Growing Herbs for Cold & Flu Relief

Excerpted from
Herbal Remedy Gardens,
by Dorie Byers

CONTENTS

Introduction

Healing with plants is not a new idea by any means. For centuries, people have used plants from their own environments to heal their ailments and to support their health. Many of these ideas, or "granny cures," as they have been called by many who now have revived their uses, were put aside in favor of more modern methods of healing early in the 20th century. Over the last two to three decades, healing with herbs has been rediscovered. This renaissance has come about with good reason, for modern research is affirming that many of the herbal treatments used through history by many cultures really do work.

If you like plants that are healing, practical, decorative, tasty, nutritious, fragrant, and otherwise useful, grow a gardenful of herbs. The word *herb* can have different meanings for different people. To me it signifies any plant that can be put to medicinal, cosmetic, culinary, decorative, or aromatic use. Gardeners often have questions about not only how to grow herbs, but how to tap into their curatives as well. I find that most are eager for this knowledge, and pleased when they learn how versatile herbs can be. Many are surprised to find that certain herbs they had not thought of as medicinal do indeed have healing properties and promote general well-being.

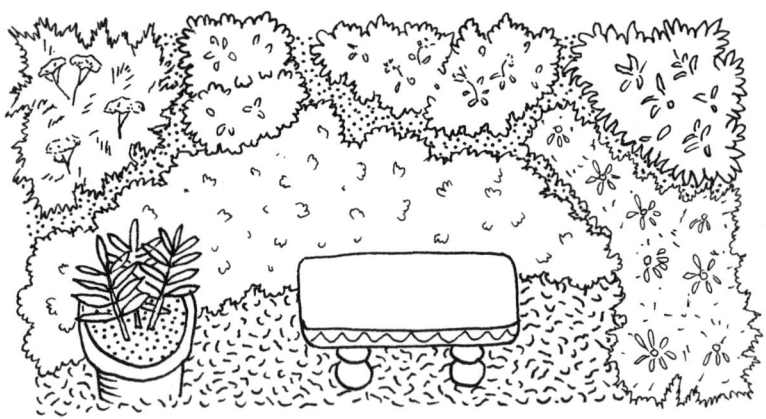

Not only will cold and flu herbs help soothe the symptoms of illness, but the garden itself can also have therapeutic benefits. Consider creating a beautiful, peaceful sanctuary by setting a small bench beside a patch of your herbs.

What Are Cold and Flu Herbs?

Each of the herbs in this bulletin is specially suited for soothing and relieving the coughs, sore throats, and congestion that come with colds and flus. Growing these herbs in your garden will help you become familiar with each one, as well as provide you with a beautiful, varied, wonderfully scented garden, plus natural remedies right at your fingertips. You'll find some recipes using these herbs here; recipes for cold and flu relief in other herbals will also call for many of these plants. So please, expand your medicine chest to include herbal teas, tinctures, infusions, and even stir-fry dishes that will chase away the symptoms that have you hiding under a blanket!

Cold and Flu Herbs

Catnip	Peppermint
Cayenne	Rosemary
Echinacea	Thyme
Garlic	Yarrow
Ginger	

Catnip (Nepeta cataria)

A member of the Mint family, this Mediterranean native was once thought to symbolize love, beauty, and happiness. In pre-Elizabethan England, people drank catnip tea in the afternoons. In fact, many gardens in colonial America included catnip.

Medicinal Uses

Commonly thought of as a treat for cats and frequently found stuffed in cat toys, this useful herb can also promote rest, improve digestion, calm and soothe stomach upsets, and relieve the symptoms of colds, flu, and fevers. It even contains antiseptic properties with which minor skin lesions can be treated. The volatile oils contained in catnip can absorb intestinal gas, so it is an age-old remedy for childhood colic. Taken before meals, it can be used to stimulate the appetite. The fresh leaves contain vitamins A, B, and C.

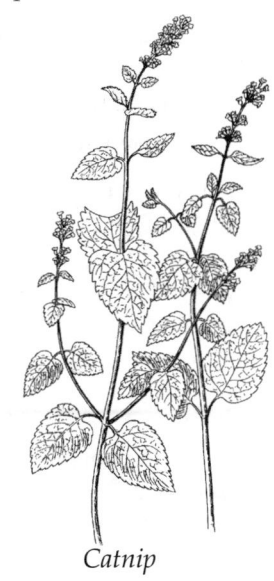

Catnip
(Nepeta cataria)

Catnip's ability to help you relax and sleep has been compared to valerian's. It is calming without being disruptive of the next day's activities.

Cautions

Catnip has many and varied uses with just one caution: You should not use catnip if you are pregnant.

🐾 CATNIP TEA 🐾

A cup of this tea in the evening hours will help you relax and prepare for sleep. Use the same infusion to alleviate cold and flu symptoms and to help settle a stomach upset from indigestion and/or gas.

> **Water**
> **1–2 teaspoons (5–10 ml) of dried herb per cup of water**

Bring the water to a boil. Place the herbs in a nonreactive container and pour the boiling water over them. Cover the container to keep the volatile oils from evaporating and let the infusion steep for 15 to 20 minutes, then strain and drink.

🐾 DECONGESTANT INHALANT 🐾

This versatile mixture is for external use only. Simmer it in a pan or place it in a reusable muslin bag for the same soothing effect.

> **Equal parts dried catnip, dried rosemary, and dried yarrow**
> **Eucalyptus essential oil**
> **A muslin tea bag**

Mix the herbs together. For each cup of dried mixture, add 4 or 5 drops of eucalyptus essential oil. Place the mixture in a muslin tea bag.

To relieve congestions, occasionally squeeze and bring this bag close to your nose to inhale. You also can place the bag on a warm register or in a sunny window to distribute the aroma into the air. Alternatively, put ¼ to ½ cup (59–118 ml) of the mixture in 1 quart (946 ml) of simmering water in a noncorrosive pan and let the aroma drift through your house.

When you're traveling, place the muslin bag on the dashboard of your car. The heat from the sun and the defroster will help disperse the aroma.

Growing Catnip

Raising catnip is easy. My first and only patch of catnip was grown from a free packet of seeds scratched into the heavy clay soil on the western side of our corrugated metal shed. There it grows year after year, spreading out some but not as drastically as its mint cousins are apt to do. It will also self-sow. The seeds germinate best when they are

planted shallowly. Further propagation can be accomplished by dividing mature plants (see box below) or by cuttings (see instructions for peppermint on page 23).

Propagation by Division

When you are growing a lot of perennial herbs, you will find that dividing them is a good way to obtain more plants. It is also a good way to renew perennial herbs that have been around for a while and are nearing the end of their usefulness.

The ideal time to divide is in spring or fall. First lift the mother plant from the soil and shake the dirt from its roots. Look at the plant for natural divisions — each new planting will need some roots and one or two stems. Pull the plant apart at those divisions, making cuts with a sharp knife or pair of scissors when necessary. Then replant each division in the soil. Water thoroughly and trim some of the top growth. Keep the new planting well watered. New growth will signal that your plant is established.

Every division should have some leaves, leaf buds, one or two stems, and roots.

The plants will thrive in well-worked, rich soil, and they enjoy moderate moisture. During dry spells, however, I rarely water my catnip plants, and they seem to get along all right. They like full sun but tolerate partial shade. The 2- to 3-foot-tall (61–91 cm) plants have gray-green leaves and clusters of white, fuzzy-looking blooms on top, which honeybees love. The plants are said to deter flea beetles, although I have never experimented with this.

Harvesting and Storing Catnip

To harvest, pick stalks of catnip before they bloom and hang them in bunches upside down from a drying rack or clothesline in a warm, dry place. Be sure that there is plenty of ventilation and room for air to circulate around the drying leaves. Once dry, strip the leaves from the stems and store in sealed glass containers in a cool, dark place. Do not crumble the leaves until you are ready to use them.

Cayenne Pepper (*Capsicum* spp.)

Grown in India, Africa, and the New World, cayenne was brought to Europe by Christopher Columbus. It was used in food preparation, and was specifically used in Africa to induce skin-cooling sweats, no doubt quite welcome in the tropical climate. The plant symbolized fidelity to some. Columbus would have been disappointed to learn that in the 17th century, European herbalists believed cayenne emitted dangerous vapors. It's not hard to see where this opinion came from, though: If someone unfamiliar with the herb takes a close whiff, it will result in reddened, watery eyes and a sharp intake of breath.

Cayenne pepper
(Capsicum annuum)

Medicinal Uses

Despite such misgivings, cayenne's uses are many. It enhances circulation, helping hot conditions cool off and cold conditions warm up. When used topically it is a counterirritant, bringing blood to the surface of the skin and causing reddening. As such, it is used to help relieve the pain of arthritic joints. Cayenne promotes digestion, increases appetite, promotes sweating, and is stimulating and energizing. Nutritionally it contains vitamins A, C, and E and is also a natural antioxidant.

Cayenne's active ingredient is capsaicin. The hotter the pepper, the more capsaicin it contains. A low concentration of capsaicin in topical creams for muscle and joint aches and pains has been available commercially the last few years. Consistent topical use four or five times a day for at least 4 weeks seems to block pain pathways to affected areas. Additional research is being done on using cayenne to treat cluster headaches.

Aside from the topical application, eating cayenne is the best way to reap its benefits. Regularly including cayenne in your diet is said to enhance your circulation and improve digestion. It will also clear up sinus congestion.

A Sure-Fire Warm-Up

For colds and chills, place ¼ to ½ teaspoon (1.3–2.5 ml) dried cayenne in 1 pint (473 ml) tomato juice and warm the mixture, stirring until the cayenne is distributed. Sip ½ to 1 cup (118–237 ml) at a time for a heat-producing, sinus-clearing, vitamin-packed drink. Store the remainder in the refrigerator for later use and rewarm before drinking.

Cautions

Always use caution when handling cayenne. Wear gloves when preparing it, keep it away from your eyes, and do not apply cayenne to damaged skin.

Cayenne is not recommended for people with active ulcers. In addition, ingesting large amounts of this herb can be harmful to the digestive tract and, possibly, the kidneys. The negative effects of

Handling the Heat

To decrease the heat of cayenne in your mouth, eat some rice or bread or drink milk; water only spreads the oil around. To remove cayenne residue from your skin, use a rinse of vinegar or milk.

cayenne on the digestive system can be counteracted, however, by eating a high protein, low-fat diet. Some people have heartburn when eating cayenne — to avoid that situation, start by adding just a pinch at a time and increase the amount to suit your palate and your stomach.

Growing Cayenne

Cayenne loves heat and full sun. One summer we toured horticultural gardens divi-ded by glass domes into different climates. In the "desert" climate grew pepper plants, which obvi-ously liked it there, because they were 3 to 4 feet (.9–1.2 m) tall and loaded with fruit. Cayenne is even toler-ant of dry conditions. In the heat of summer, when the rest of your plants are wilting, the cayenne pepper plants will still be going strong.

Growing at a Glance

OPTIMAL GROWING CONDITIONS:
Warm to hot soil and air temperatures

ZONES:
5 to 10 with lots of sun and heat; cayenne is hardy in Zone 10

COMMON PROPAGATION:
Seeds, transplants

TYPE OF PLANT:
Annual

I like to start my peppers in early spring so that strong plants can move outside in late spring. Presprouting seeds seems to work the best for me. To presprout, place the seeds in a single layer on a damp paper towel, roll up the paper towel, and place it in a resealable plastic bag. You can put this on top of the hot water heater, heat register, or any other place consistently warm. Check the seeds after a couple of days and every day thereafter. When they have started to sprout, plant them shallowly in containers with damp, sterile potting mix. Place in a warm spot that receives 16 hours of strong light a day.

Transplant cayenne into your garden after all danger of frost is past. These heat lovers would never survive a frost. Ideally, pepper plants should not be transplanted until the soil temperature reaches 65°F (18°C) 4 inches (10 cm) belowground. The plants themselves will grow into "bushes" that are 2 to 3 feet (61–91 cm) tall and 3 feet (91 cm) in diameter with 3- to 6-inch-long (8–15 cm) slender, slightly curved fruits that are green and turn red when ripe. The redder the fruits, the higher their vitamin content.

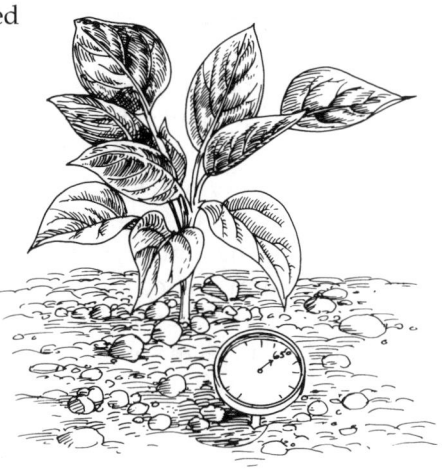

Transplant cayenne seedlings when the soil has warmed up — ideally to 65°F (18°C)— and all danger of frost has passed.

Harvesting and Storing Cayenne

To harvest, pick the ripe red fruits with their stems on. Thread the fruits on heavy string or fishing line, piercing the stems only, and hang this in a warm place out of direct sun until dry.

After they are dry, you can store the peppers whole or grind them into powder in your food processor. Use care when doing this, for pepper dust in the air can be quite irritating to your senses. Do not remove the cover from your food processor until all of the dust has settled. Store the dried cayenne in a glass jar away from heat and light.

Echinacea (Echinacea purpurea, E. angustifolia, and E. pallida)

Commonly known as the purple coneflower, the name "echinacea" seems to be on everyone's lips these days, and it is widely touted in print as well. Best known for their ability to boost the immune system, echinacea pills fill the shelves of health-food stores as well as drugstores. The plant is well known not only by people familiar with herbs but also by those who aren't usually in the "herbal know."

Medicinal Uses

Native Americans, who had been using the plant to treat snakebites, fevers, wounds, and poisonous insect bites for generations, taught the European settlers how to use echinacea. In the 1880s, a pharmaceutical manufacturer in the United States started to sell different forms of echinacea. By the 1920s it was the country's most popular medicinal plant, but it lost favor when new and effective synthetic medicines appeared.

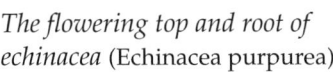

The flowering top and root of echinacea (Echinacea purpurea)

Commission E, a special committee of the German Federal Department of Health, reviews the effects of herbs and their safety and publishes the results. It has approved echinacea for combating recurring infections and as a local application for treatment of hard-to-heal wounds. This latter use has been justified by studies that show an accelerated healing rate of bacterial skin infections when echinacea is applied.

The plant's other properties include antiseptic, antimicrobial, lymphatic, and tonic. Usually echinacea's root is the part used, although the aerial part of the plant has been used successfully in some preparations. By and large echinacea is best known for its ability to stimulate and/or support the body's immune system against bacterial and viral attacks. At the first sign of cold or flu, start taking echinacea — the tinctured form is the most reliable. Take doses of echinacea during waking hours for 2 days, then stop. It is meant to be taken only as an immune-system booster — not on a regular basis. Echinacea will not cure a cold or flu if you take it after the illness has taken hold.

Cautions for Echinacea

Echinacea should be used with caution by pregnant women. In addition, do not use echinacea if you suffer from any of the following conditions:

- an allergy to sunflowers
- a severe systemic immune disorder such as multiple sclerosis or tuberculosis
- a collagen disease such as lupus or scleroderma

❧ ECHINACEA TINCTURE ❧

*Echinacea's active ingredients aren't all water soluble; a tincture is the
best way to obtain its benefits.*

- ¾ **cup (177 ml) pure grain alcohol** or **80 to 100 proof (40 to 50%
  alcohol) vodka or brandy** or **glycerin**
- ¾ **cup (177 ml) distilled water**
- 1½ **ounces (42 g) echinacea root, chopped**

To make:

1. Combine the alcohol with the distilled water in
a jar with a tight-fitting lid.

2. Add the echinacea root. Run a knife or chop-
stick around the edges of the jar to release any
trapped air bubbles.

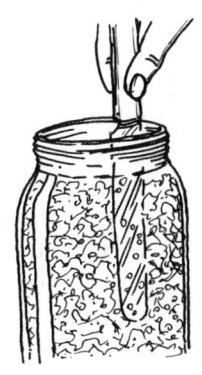

Step 2

3. Replace the lid and set the jar in a cool, dark
place for 2 weeks. Shake the mixture every day.

4. Strain the mixture to remove the herb. This
must be done quickly or the alcohol will evaporate. I usually pour the mixture into a strainer
lined with an unbleached paper coffee filter and
place it in the refrigerator as it strains, to slow the
evaporation of the alcohol. After straining,
squeeze the filter to remove as much of the liquid
as possible.

5. Store the tincture in a tightly sealed glass container in a cool, dark
location, where it will keep for up to 5 years. Be sure to label the
bottle first!

To use:

At the first sign of cold or flu's onset, herbal experts recommend
30 drops of tincture every 3 hours for the first 2 days only. Once you
have developed a full-blown case of a cold or flu, echinacea probably
will not cure it.

If you are unable to take the alcohol in the tincture, add the tincture to a small glass of warm water and stir gently. The warm water
will cause the alcohol to evaporate.

Growing Echinacea

Growing your own echinacea is a good idea, since it is being harvested to extinction in the wild. Very little effort is needed to grow echinacea, but the seeds do need to be stratified. I put them into damp vermiculite in a resealable plastic bag. Then I put the bag in the refrigerator

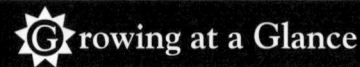

Growing at a Glance

OPTIMAL GROWING CONDITIONS:
   Full sun, warm to hot soil

ZONES:
   3 to 9

COMMON PROPAGATION:
   Seeds, division

TYPE OF PLANT:
   Perennial

for a month. After that time, I plant the seeds in flats and place under grow lights in a warm place. In less than a week, my seeds will have sprouted. When the weather outside has settled and danger of frost has passed, transplant the seedlings outside. The plants will grow slowly at first, and they probably will not bloom the first year.

If you want flowers the first year, mature echinacea plants can be divided and transplanted. They are available from local nurseries and by mail order. Echinacea multiplies readily, and neighborly gardeners may give you a division. Echinacea prefers a sunny location. It is even happy on the southern side of my house right next to the bricks, which soak up a lot of heat in the summer. It grows to about 3 feet (91 cm) in height and will spread gradually as far as you let it.

The petals of the flowers are a mauve color with orange-brown centers. When the plant blooms, expect a wonderful show of butter-flies. When the blossoms are finished, they will dry out and reseed themselves in your flower and herb beds; remove the spent blooms if you don't want this to occur.

Harvesting and Storing Echinacea

To harvest echinacea, dig the roots after the plant has bloomed — usually in early fall. Only harvest 2- to 4-year-old roots, making sure that you leave enough plants for future use and propagation. Wash and dry the roots thoroughly, then chop them coarsely. Store the dried roots in a tightly covered glass container and keep away from direct heat and light.

Garlic (*Allium sativum*)

Because this plant has been around for millennia, it is difficult to know where to start when discussing garlic. It's one of the oldest-known cultivated herbs. The Egyptians believed that it prevented illness and increased strength and endurance. It is even rumored that the workers who built the pyramids ate garlic to sustain them in their labors.

Greek athletes ate garlic before participating in races, and Greek soldiers ate garlic before battle. When the Romans conquered Gaul, they brought garlic with them. Nowadays garlic, also known as the stinking rose, is believed to help alleviate many ailments. It's also said to symbolize protection and healing. Perhaps that is why, in folklore, it is believed that wearing a garland of garlic will protect you from vampires.

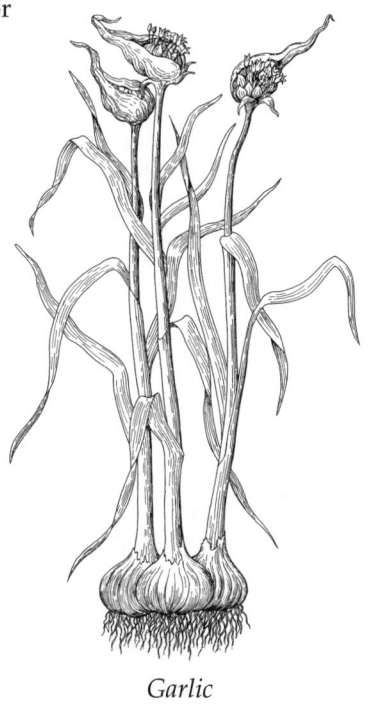

Garlic
(Allium sativum)

Medicinal Uses

Garlic's properties include antiseptic, antiviral, diaphoretic, cholagogue, hypotensive, and antispasmodic. It has sulfur-containing compounds, enzymes, B vitamins, minerals, and flavonoids. In its raw form garlic can act on bacteria, viruses, and alimentary parasites. For this reason it can be used as a preventive in many infectious conditions. The volatile oils that give garlic its scent are excreted by the lungs and through the skin.

The best news on garlic seems to be its effect on the cardiovascular system. Studies have suggested that, with regular use, garlic helps reduce blood cholesterol levels and blood pressure. This has helped to make garlic a best-seller in the vitamin and supplement world today. To lower cholesterol, you must eat the equivalent of two cloves a day.

Other positive studies imply that garlic may help AIDS patients by increasing killer-cell activity and possibly inhibiting malignant-cell formation. The downside to all of this news is that garlic can cause heartburn in susceptible people. Additionally, its odor is offensive to some individuals. (If you're concerned about odor, there are deodorized garlic preparations available.)

The best way to take garlic is by eating it. There are many wonderful recipes that include this flavorful bulb — keep in mind that it is most effective when eaten raw. Cutting or crushing the cloves before eating them allows garlic to be more effective, because its active ingredients are released readily into your system. If you are concerned about your breath, chew some fresh parsley after eating garlic.

Cautions for Garlic

Garlic can thin the blood, so avoid using it if you are already taking blood thinners or before surgery. The use of garlic other than in culinary amounts during pregnancy and nursing is not recommended. In addition, excessive topical use of this herb can cause irritation.

⬤ GARLICKY HERBAL BROTH ⬤

This flavorful, warming broth is packed full of vitamins.

    6   minced garlic cloves
    1   tablespoon (15 ml) olive oil
    2   cups (473 ml) water or vegetable broth
    1   teaspoon (5 ml) finely chopped fresh cayenne pepper, or
         ½ teaspoon (2.5 ml) dried powdered cayenne
    1   teaspoon (5 ml) finely chopped fresh rosemary, or ½ teaspoon
         (2.5 ml) dried
    ½   teaspoon (2.5 ml) fresh thyme, or ¼ teaspoon (1.3 ml) dried
    A pinch of salt, if the vegetable broth is unsalted

1. In a large saucepan, combine the garlic and olive oil and sauté over high heat briefly, until the garlic starts to change color.

2. Add the broth or water, turn down the heat to medium-low, and simmer for 20 minutes.

3. Add all of the herbs and salt to taste. Simmer for 5 more minutes, then serve. Sip slowly.

Growing Garlic

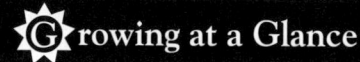

There are two types of garlic that you can grow, depending on your location. Soft-neck varieties are the most productive; these are the ones found in grocery stores. They like mild winters and store very well. This is the garlic that is most commonly seen braided. Hard-neck types like cold winters and

OPTIMAL GROWING CONDITIONS:
Rich soil, long growing season

ZONES:
5 to 10; hard-neck varieties can possibly grow in Zones 3 and 4

COMMON PROPAGATION:
Cloves

TYPE OF PLANT:
Annual

are the best choice for areas that have changing seasons.

I've found that garlic can be somewhat tricky to grow. In fall, about 6 weeks before the ground freezes, separate the cloves from the bulb and plant them, pointed end up, about 1 inch (2.5 cm) deep and 4 to 6 inches (10–15 cm) apart, into rich, well-worked soil. This is important: If your soil is heavy clay and/or stripped of its nutrients, you will end up with a harvest of puny garlic bulbs. After the first freeze, mulch the site to protect the soil from heaving and evicting the bulbs from their growing place.

Plant the cloves with their pointed ends up and flat basal plates down.

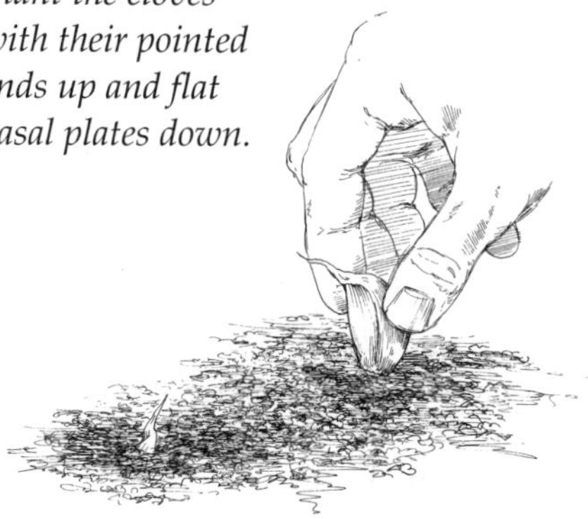

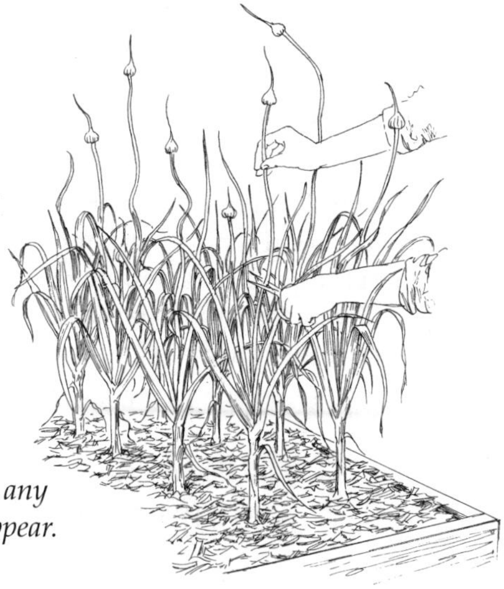

As the plants grow, trim any flower stalks that may appear.

In spring after the weather has settled, remove the mulch. Your garlic cloves should be sprouting green foliage that is wider and more strappy than that of onions. The plants will grow throughout the summer. During the first month or two, they will appreciate a good watering once a week from you if nature doesn't provide it. In late spring some varieties may send up flower stalks — trim these so that the plants can keep their energy directed into forming large bulbs.

Harvesting and Storing Garlic

Near the end of summer or early fall, bend over the tops of the plants to encourage drying. When the tops start to shrivel, harvest the bulbs. Don't let them get too brown; this is a sign that the bulbs are rotting. Cure, or dry, the bulbs under warm, dry conditions.

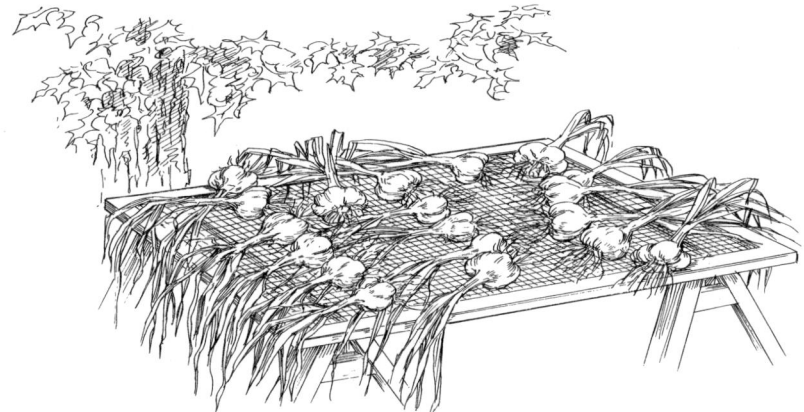

A window screen set on sawhorses makes a good platform for drying garlic.

The bulbs will store best in cool (not cold), dry conditions. I have found that the small ceramic storage pots with holes in the top that are specially designed for garlic (available at kitchen-supply stores) provide great storage conditions at room temperature.

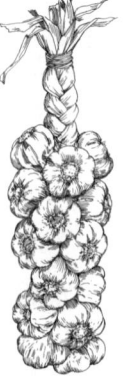

Braiding the bulbs is both a classic and a space-efficient way to store garlic.

Ginger (*Zingiber officinale*)

In the United States, ginger is commonly thought of as a baking spice. For the last few years, though, the fresh root has also been available in Asian dishes, giving them a warm to hot, distinctively spicy flavor. I have come to enjoy this tropical rhizome so much that I keep it on hand to use and have even started growing it.

Ginger was prominent in Chinese herbal practices circa 3000 B.C., and in India ginger has been widely used in Ayurvedic medicine. The herb was brought to Europe via the trade routes from the Far East, and Spanish conquistadors brought the herb to the New World via Jamaica.

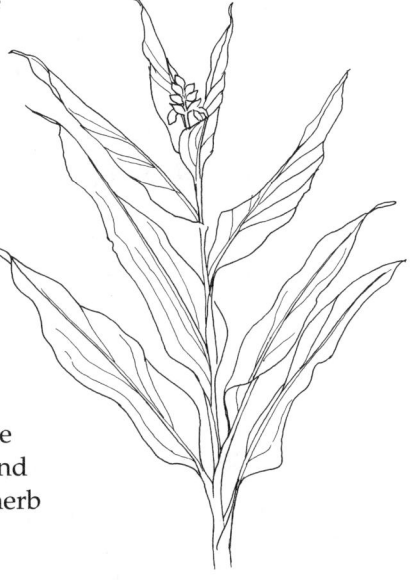

Ginger
(Zingiber officinale)

Medicinal Uses

Nowadays, fresh ginger is becoming more popular in our country. It is rich in volatile oils whose properties include stimulant, anti-spasmodic, anti-inflammatory, carminative, rubefacient, and dia-phoretic. The spicy rhizome also contains powerful antioxidant properties. Ginger's actions on the digestive tract are notable. It works indirectly to increase the availability of dietary nutrients for digestion and metabolism. It promotes the gastric secretions that aid in digestion of food. Ginger is also a gastrointestinal tract stimulant. While it will aid in relieving nausea and indigestion from various causes, it can also reduce the nausea associated with motion sickness; some studies have found ginger to be superior to pharmacological substances in this.

> ### Quick Tip
>
> To ease symptoms of motion sickness when traveling, take ginger at the first sign of queasiness. Try incorporating it fresh into a small snack or drinking a cup of ginger tea.

Ginger is also stimulating to the peripheral circulation, making it a good topically applied treatment for minor muscle aches and pains. It relaxes peripheral blood vessels, bringing blood to the skin's surface and causing a counterirritant. Taken as a tea, ginger can help to alleviate cold and flu discomfort, including sinus congestion. For feverish conditions, it can promote perspiration.

Cautions for Ginger

Although culinary use during pregnancy is all right, larger quantities of ginger during pregnancy are not recommended. Avoid excessive intake if you suffer from peptic ulcers. Ginger may raise blood pressure, so avoid it if this is a problem for you. Ginger may increase the activities of blood-thinning drugs.

🍲 DUAL-PURPOSE GINGER STIR-FRY 🍲

Have some of this recipe to both please your palate and help give you relief from congestion. This can be served as a side dish or over rice for a vegetarian main course. And though this recipe can help kick a cold out the door, you don't have to be congested to enjoy it!

> Nonstick cooking spray or 1 teaspoon (5 ml) vegetable oil
> 6   cups (1.4 l) cabbage cut into 4-inch (10 cm) slices
> 1   tablespoon (15 ml) fresh ginger, grated
> ¼   cup (59 ml) water
> A pinch of cayenne
> A pinch of salt

1. Spray a saucepan with nonstick cooking spray, or coat the surface with about 1 teaspoon (5 ml) of vegetable oil. Place the pan on your stovetop over high heat; add the cabbage and ginger and sauté in the oil for a couple of minutes, stirring frequently.

2. Pour the water over the cabbage. Stir and cook the cabbage until it is crisp-tender, 10 to 15 minutes.

3. Turn the stovetop heat down to medium-low. Add the cayenne and salt; stir the seasonings into the cabbage. Serve immediately.

Growing Ginger

True to its nature as a tropical plant, ginger enjoys heat and moisture. To grow ginger, buy a firm rhizome (also known as gingerroot) at the grocery store. Avoid the rhizomes that are shriveled and/or moldy. Have a container 10 to 12 inches (25–30 cm) wide prepared with a potting mixture that facilitates good drainage. Place the rhizome about 1 inch (2.5 cm) deep into the mix. You can place the rhizome with its flat side parallel to the top of the potting mixture or perpendicular to the bottom of the container. It seems to grow equally well either way.

Place the container in a warm, partially shady situation and keep the soil continuously moist. I like to fill the dish the container is sitting in with water, and refill this as the moisture is taken up by the contents of the container. Be patient — the rhizomes take quite some time to sprout. Put the container outside in the warm months, taking care to provide continuous moisture and partial shade. You will

☼Growing at a Glance

OPTIMAL GROWING CONDITIONS:
Hot, moist

ZONES:
9 and 10; in growing zones farther north, you must grow ginger in containers and take them inside with the onset of cold weather

COMMON PROPAGATION:
Rhizomes

TYPE OF PLANT:
Tender perennial

be rewarded with a thriving tropical plant after a few weeks. Ginger will even bloom given the right conditions. I have not been fortunate enough to achieve this,although I know people who have been so lucky.

Harvesting and Storing Ginger

Ginger is best used fresh. To harvest, dig up the rhizome no earlier than 9 weeks after it started growing, cut or break off what you need, and replant what is left. Peeled fresh ginger can be used chopped up or grated. The root can be wrapped and frozen for future use.

Peppermint (*Mentha x piperita*)

Peppermint appeared as a sterile crossbreed in the late 1600s in England, so any history of the plant starts there. However, the mint cousins, such as spearmint and watermint, from which it derived have been around through the ages. The Egyptian Pharisees paid tithes to the pharaoh with mint; in the early medical record known as Egyptian Ebers Papyrus of 1550 B.C., it was recommended that mint tea be used to alleviate indigestion. In Greece soldiers rubbed their weapons with mint before battle for good luck. The Romans chewed mint after meals, and, as with other herbs that they used, took it with them when they moved, thus spreading mint to other parts of the world.

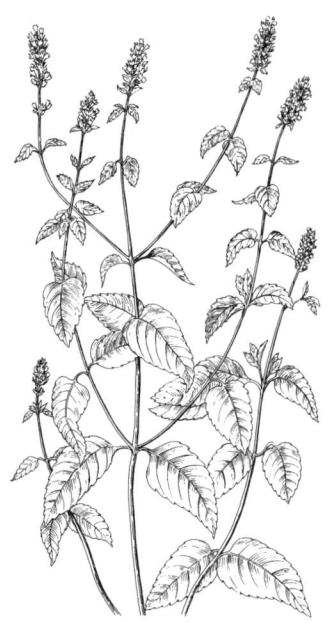

In early Christian times the herb was such a valuable medicine that the Church accepted it as a payment of tithes. Medieval Europeans used it as a strewing herb and rubbed it on their teeth for fresh breath. They also used the herb to relieve toothaches. Colonists in North America grew mint in their gardens, and there it has grown ever since.

Peppermint (Mentha x piperita)

Medicinal Uses

Peppermint's useful properties include carminative, antispasmodic, aromatic, diaphoretic, antiseptic, analgesic, and nervine. Peppermint's volatile oil contains menthol, an ingredient that is familiar to us in many products. It is known to relax visceral muscles. Peppermint contains calcium, vitamins A and C, and riboflavin. The aroma encourages alertness and wakefulness.

You can use peppermint infusions, or teas (see recipe on the facing page), to relieve a variety of digestive-tract ailments; they stimulate bile production, thereby enhancing digestive activity. They will also help relieve gas and accompanying abdominal pain. The volatile oil acts as a mild anesthetic to the stomach wall, helping decrease nausea and vomiting. Externally, peppermint stimulates cold-perceiving nerves below the surface of the skin. It can relieve itching and be useful for easing achy muscles.

Cautions for Peppermint

Although peppermint is a wonderful medicinal herb and is safe for use by almost everyone, there are a couple of cautions:

- Those suffering from anemia should be careful, because large amounts of peppermint tea can inhibit the absorption of iron in severely anemic people and can also be toxic.
- Don't give peppermint tea to babies and small children — the volatile oils can cause them to have a choking sensation.

❧ PEPPERMINT TEA ❧

1   cup (237 ml) boiling water
1   tablespoon (15 ml) fresh chopped peppermint or 1 teaspoon (5 ml) dried

Pour the boiling water over the peppermint. Cover and let steep for 10 to 20 minutes.

❧ PEPPERMINT INHALATION ❧

When suffering from congestion due to a cold and/or a sinus condition, peppermint can be helpful simmered in water as an inhalation.

1   quart (946 ml) water
½   cup dried (118 ml) or 1 cup (237 ml) fresh peppermint

Combine the water and peppermint in an enamel or stainless-steel saucepan. Bring to a boil, reduce heat, and allow to simmer, uncovered, on the stovetop; this will release the peppermint aroma into the air. You will enjoy greater benefits if you are in the same room as the mixture.

An alternative way to prepare the inhalation is in a small simmering potpourri pot, which is more portable and can be placed in any room you choose. Do not allow the mixture to boil dry; add more water if needed.

Growing Peppermint

The very phrase "growing peppermint" is a gross misstatement, given peppermint's propensity to take off. Like its other mint relatives, once peppermint is planted in a favorable area, it will grow and spread to an amazing degree. The first year I planted mine, it went from one tiny stem to a 1½-foot (46 cm) clump. The next year it grew to a patch about 4 feet around.

Beware of any packages of seeds that claim to be peppermint; this plant is sterile, which means it cannot be started from seed. Instead, you must start it from cuttings (see below) or division (see page 5). You'll want to contain it, somehow — perhaps by planting it in a large container that you sink into the ground. I let all of my mints grow as they will, taking a shovel or garden fork and digging out clumps around the edges to contain them. These clumps can be easily divided and potted up for plant or garage sales or for hands-on lessons for gardening students learning to divide plants.

Peppermint will grow in very moist conditions without complaint. Its light requirements are sun to partial shade. The plant has attractive purplish stems that grow to be 18 to 30 inches (45–76 cm) tall. Its lavender blooms appear in late summer.

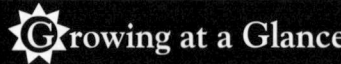

Growing at a Glance

OPTIMAL GROWING CONDITIONS:
Moist and rich soil, sun to partial shade

ZONES:
4 to 10; may be grown as an annual in Zone 3 or brought in as a container plant

COMMON PROPAGATION:
Division, cuttings

TYPE OF PLANT:
Perennial

Harvesting and Storing Peppermint

To harvest peppermint, cut the stems and dry the leaves while still attached. Ideally you'll do this before the plants bloom. When they are dry, use your fingers to strip the leaves from the stems, and store in a glass container away from heat and light.

Growing Peppermint from a Cutting

The best time to take cuttings from peppermint plants is from early spring to late fall. First prepare a clean container and a light seed-starting mix. With a sharp pair of scissors, snip 3 to 6 inches from the top of a peppermint plant, cutting just above a leaf node. Trim the bottom of the cutting to just below its bottommost leaf node, strip off its lower leaves, and remove any blooms. Insert the lower half of the cutting into the potting medium and carefully firm the mix around the stem.

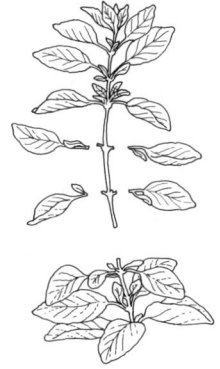

Place the cutting in a warm spot out of direct sunlight. Lightly mist it twice a day with room-temperature water. Do not overwater — the soil should be kept damp but not water-logged. You will know that the cutting has taken root when the plant resists being pulled up with gentle tugging and there is new top growth. It may take several weeks for this to happen, so be patient!

Strip off the lower leaves before transplanting the cutting.

Rosemary (*Rosmarinus* spp.)

Greek students wore rosemary in garlands on their heads when they were taking exams; they felt that it improved their memory. Medieval households used rosemary-scented water for hand washing. It was believed that rosemary refused to grow in gardens of evil people, an idea that is disconcerting to me, given that there have been some years when I can't keep a single plant alive! In the Middle Ages people carried sprigs of rosemary in their pockets to ward off evil spirits and placed sprigs under their pillows to prevent nightmares.

Rosemary has been burned in sick chambers to purify the air, and branches were strewn in law courts to protect those present from jail fever, also known as

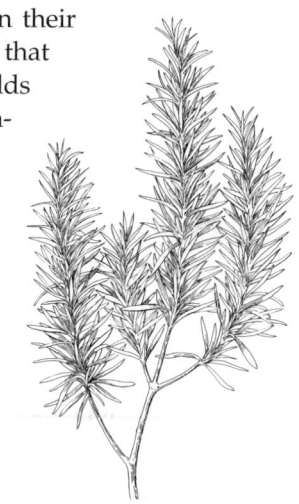

Rosemary
(Rosmarinus officinalis)

typhus. Likewise, during the Middle Ages it was believed that the reason rosemary flowers are blue is that the Virgin Mary laid her blue cloak across a rosemary bush when it was in bloom, coloring the flowers. The herb was woven into bridal wreaths as a symbol of fidelity and constancy. Rosemary's natural antioxidant properties, which slow food spoilage, made it appropriate for food preservation in the days before refrigeration.

Medicinal Uses

Rosemary contains antioxidant, antiviral, carminative, antibacterial, anti-inflammatory, and circulatory stimulant properties. Recent research has shown that rosemary enhances the cells' intake of oxygen, which aids in cerebral function. Rosemary contains calcium, magnesium, phosphorus, sodium, potassium, and vitamins A and C.

STIMULATING ROSEMARY BATH

For a stimulating soak that will relieve a tired, achy body, add a rosemary infusion to your bath or footbath!

1   **cup (237 ml) dried rosemary**
2   **quarts (1.9 l) boiling water**

Pour the boiling water over the rosemary. Cover and let steep for 10 minutes, then strain. For a footbath, add the infusion to a basin of warm water. For a full bath, add the infusion to a warm tub.

ROSEMARY-GINGER TEA

Here is something warm and aromatic for you to sip while you lounge around in your bunny slippers, recuperating from the tiring effects of a cold or the flu.

1   **cup (237 ml) boiling water**
1   **tablespoon (15 ml) fresh ginger, grated**
1   **teaspoon (5 ml) dried rosemary, or 2 teaspoons (10 ml) fresh**
Honey (optional)

Pour the boiling water over the ginger and rosemary. Cover the mixture and let steep for 10 to 20 minutes. Strain, add honey to taste, and sip slowly.

Cautions for Rosemary

Due to its stimulating properties, rosemary should be used as an internal infusion for a maximum of 2 cups a day for no longer than a week at a time. In addition, people with high blood pressure should avoid rosemary in other than culinary uses.

Growing Rosemary

There are several ways to grow rosemary. One is by taking cuttings (see description for peppermint on page 23); another is to layer a low-lying stem into the soil where the plant is growing (see box on the next page). While these two methods work best for all varieties of rosemary, with a little care common rosemary, or *Rosmarinus officinalis*, can be started from seeds: After

☀ Growing at a Glance

OPTIMAL GROWING CONDITIONS:
Medium to rich well-drained soil, warm temperatures

ZONES:
8 to 10; in other zones, treat rosemary as an annual or place in containers for wintering indoors

COMMON PROPAGATION:
Cuttings

TYPE OF PLANT:
Tender perennial

barely covering the seeds with starting mix, mist the soil daily to prevent a crust from forming over them. Plant more seeds than you will want plants, for the germination rate is low. After the seedlings have emerged, continue misting them.

Rosemary is tender and will not survive outdoors in areas that receive frost. To keep it alive, take cuttings to raise indoors, or dig up plants from the ground and move to pots when temperatures turn cool.

Allow container-grown rosemary to dry out between waterings. The plants will enjoy a daily misting, particularly in homes with low humidity. A lot of people think their rosemary is dead when the leaves resemble those of a parched Christmas tree. My answer is to water the plant and wait a day to see what happens. Chances are good that it will perk up.

Harvesting and Storing Rosemary

To harvest rosemary, cut off the stems and allow the leaves to become crumbly dry. Strip the leaves from the stems into a glass container; seal and place away from light or heat.

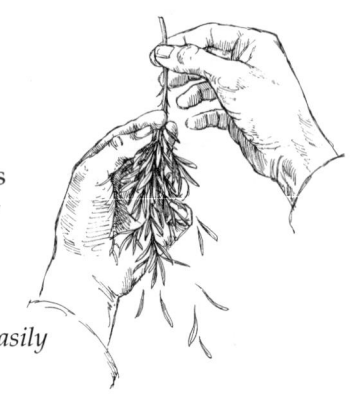

Once dried, rosemary leaves can be easily stripped from their stems.

Propagation by Layering

Layering your plants requires less equipment and time than any other propagation method. The new plant forms while still attached to the mother plant, so the stem still obtains food and life strength from its plant of origin.

In spring, summer, or fall, select from the outer part of the mother plant a stem that will easily bend and touch the ground. Strip away any leaves from the section of the stem that touches the soil, then take a knife and scrape away (or "wound") the outer coating of the stem at that spot. Dig and loosen the soil where the stem section touches. Anchor the stem to the ground using wire pins and bury the wounded section an inch or two into the soil. You can also stake the stem to a small stick. Water well. When roots have formed — 6 to 8 weeks in spring or summer, the next spring in fall — cut the layered stem from the mother plant. If desired, you can then uproot the new plant and move it to another spot in the garden.

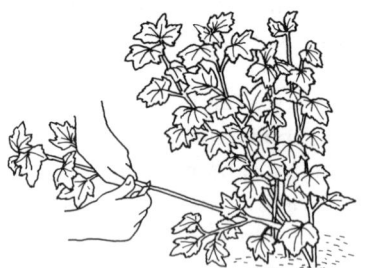

Wound the selected stem at the spot where it touches the soil.

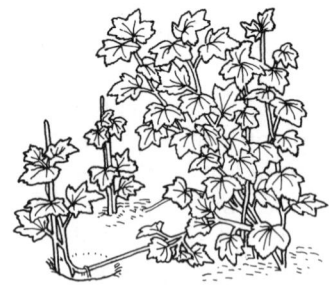

Anchor the wounded stem to the ground until new roots form.

Thyme *(Thymus vulgaris)*

The ancient Greek physician Hippocrates and his contemporaries prized thyme highly for its medicinal qualities. In Greece a supreme compliment was to say that someone "smelled of thyme." It was burned as incense in ancient Greek temples. In ancient Rome thyme was burned as a deodorizer, and Roman soldiers bathed in it for vigor. The Egyptians used it medicinally, too. The Crusaders brought the seeds home with them, and thyme became a common addition to their families' gardens and households. Early Europeans used the herb for strewing and to make an infusion that combated excessive body lice.

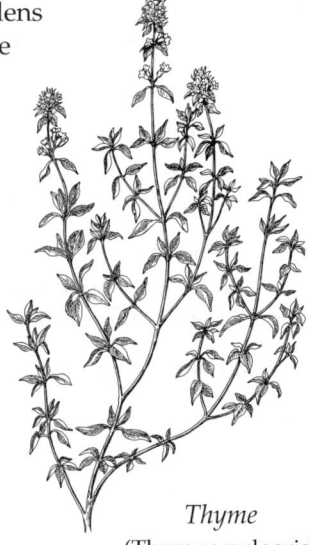

Thyme
(Thymus vulgaris)

Thyme's essential oil is strongly antiseptic, and during World War I it was used for that reason. Throughout various periods in history thyme has been used for such diverse complaints as colic, melancholia, sore throat, insomnia, nightmares, hangovers, and alcohol addiction. Thyme symbolizes health, healing, sleep, psychic powers, love, purification, and courage.

Medicinal Uses

Thyme's properties are carminative, antimicrobial, antispasmodic, expectorant, stimulant, relaxant, and astringent. Research done in Japan shows that thyme works as an antioxidant as well. It contains vitamins A and D, niacin, phosphorus, potassium, calcium, iron, magnesium, and zinc.

Thyme's best medicinal use, in my opinion, is as an adjunct in treating sore throats, colds, and congestion. An infusion, or tea, made from the herb (see page 28) will help soothe a sore throat and act as an expectorant, due to an active constituent found in thyme called thymol. German studies have found thyme to be effective for the treatment of symptoms of bronchitis, coughs, and colds.

Thyme's antimicrobial property makes it a good choice for use in skin care. A cool infusion, or tea, of the leaves and flowers can be used as a facial lotion for blemished skin.

✿ THYME TEA ✿

1   cup (237 ml) boiling water
1   teaspoon (5 ml) dried thyme, or 2 teaspoons (10 ml) fresh
Honey

Pour the boiling water over the thyme. Cover and steep the infusion for 10 to 20 minutes, then strain. Adding honey increases the infusion's effectiveness.

✿ THYME-INFUSED HONEY ✿

This is a most pleasant way to ingest thyme when you're suffering from a cold and congestion.

1   cup (237 ml) honey
½   cup (118 ml) fresh thyme, or ¼ cup (59 ml) dried

1. Combine the two ingredients in a saucepan and heat gently over low heat for 15 to 20 minutes, making sure the honey does not boil or scorch. Remove from the heat and allow the honey to cool.

2. Strain out the herbs, then bottle the honey and label it.

To use: To relieve colds, coughs, and sore throats, take 1 teaspoon (5 ml) of honey three times a day. You can also add a teaspoon to a cup of regular hot tea and sip slowly.

Cautions

Do not give thyme preparations to children under the age of 3. In addition, avoid all but culinary uses of thyme if you:

- have thyroid problems
- have high blood pressure
- are pregnant

Growing Thyme

There is a multitude of thyme varieties of different aromas, heights, and foliage colors, which makes thyme a good plant to include in garden planning. For optimal use of thyme's healing properties, however, the common thyme *(Thymus vulgaris)* is the best choice. Thyme is low growing and makes a nice border for a garden. People used to plant it for the fairies to live under, and no wonder: It is just the right size for them!

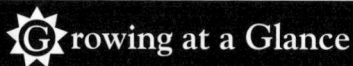

Starting common thyme from seeds is trouble-free. Plant the seeds indoors in early spring, barely covering them, and give them an environment of around 70°F (21°C) in which to germinate. Mist the top of the soil to keep it moist and prevent crusting over. Transplant the seedlings when the weather is warm and the danger of heavy frost is past. Give thyme a sunny spot with well-drained soil in which to grow and you will be rewarded with 8- to 12-inch-tall (20–30cm) plants that will expand to about 12 inches (30 cm) high, looking like little shrubs. The tiny, prolific, pale lavender flowers are quite beautiful and will attract bees to your garden to help pollinate your plants. Thyme will stay green in all but the coldest months of winter, and it will never need watering, not even in the driest months of summer.

This herb can also be propagated by cuttings (see page 23) and layering (see page 26). Often the lowermost branches will touch the ground and layer themselves, giving you starts for additional plants. This season I even had some thyme self-seed; I found new little seedlings sprouting in the cracks of the stepping-stones in my garden. Thyme can be grown in containers and brought in for winter availability of the fresh herb. It does tend to get leggy when grown indoors.

Harvesting and Storing Thyme

Thyme's active properties are at their peak just as the plant is coming into bloom. To harvest, cut the stems about halfway down and dry them. Strip the leaves and flowers and store in a tightly covered glass container away from heat and light.

Yarrow (*Achillea millefolium*)

Yarrow is said to be named for the ancient hero Achilles, who was supposed to have used the herb to treat his wounded soldiers. Yarrow was indeed a popular wound treatment for the ancient Greeks, and continued to be popular into the mid-19th century, when it was used by field doctors in the American Civil War. Native Americans used yarrow to halt bleeding and promote wound healing. It's not known whether European settlers introduced yarrow to the New World or if it is native to North America. Nevertheless, it is quite a useful plant.

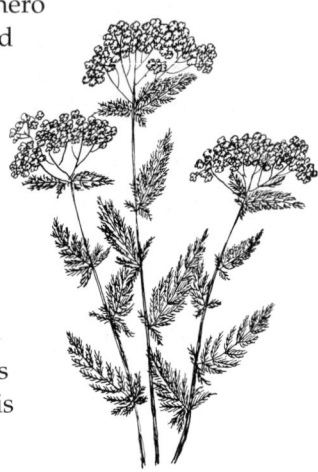

Yarrow
(Achillea millefolium)

Medicinal Uses

Yarrow's properties are diaphoretic, hypotensive, astringent, antiseptic, hemostatic, and anti-inflammatory, and it was traditionally used to treat wounds. To treat a minor cut or scrape that is bleeding, take a clean leaf or two of yarrow, crush it, and apply to the wound. The hemostatic and antiseptic properties should help to stop the bleeding and promote healing. Its diaphoretic property gives yarrow infusions the reputation of being helpful in feverish conditions.

BREATHE-FREE HERBAL INHALER

The aromas from this herbal infusion will aid in clearing your stuffy nose.

> 2   quarts (1.9 l) water
> ¼   cup (59 ml) fresh yarrow, or 2 tablespoons (30 ml) dried
> ¼   cup fresh (59 ml) peppermint, or 2 tablespoons (30 ml) dried
> 1   tablespoon (15 ml) fresh rosemary, or 2 teaspoons (10 ml) dried
> 1   tablespoon (15 ml) fresh thyme, or 2 teaspoons (10 ml) dried

Place the water in a saucepan on the stove. Add all of the herbs. Simmer, uncovered, over low heat for 30 to 45 minutes. This allows the herbal essences to drift through the house.

Caution: Do not allow the contents to boil dry.

❧ YARROW INFUSION ❧

1   cup (237 ml) boiling water
1   teaspoon (5 ml) dried yarrow, or 2 teaspoons (10 ml) fresh

Pour the boiling water over the yarrow. Cover and let steep for 10 to 20 minutes. Sip slowly. Drink no more than 3 cups (711 ml) of the infusion a day.

Cautions

As with all herbs, moderation is in order. Consider the following precautions:

- Taking too much yarrow over a prolonged period can cause headaches and vertigo.
- Prolonged use of yarrow can interfere with the absorption of iron and other minerals.
- When combined with other herbs, yarrow can intensify their medicinal actions — consult a qualified herbal practitioner before you decide to take it regularly.
- Prolonged use of yarrow can make the skin light-sensitive.
- Yarrow is a member of the Daisy family, so do not use it if you have related allergies.
- Yarrow should not be ingested if you are pregnant.

Growing Yarrow

If you look around your property, you may realize that you don't need to raise yarrow. Regarded as a weed by many people, it may already be on your land somewhere. Move it to a place where you would like to have it growing. If you don't already have yarrow, it is easy to start. It is very hardy and likes full sun. It will

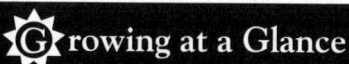

Growing at a Glance

OPTIMAL GROWING CONDITIONS:
   Full sun, poor to moderate soil

ZONES:
   3 to 9

COMMON PROPAGATION:
   Seeds, division

TYPE OF PLANT:
   Perennial

grow in poor soils as well as rich, and is very drought tolerant. Plant the seeds in a spot with full sun after the soil has warmed. Cover them lightly with a little soil. Soon you will see little plants with the characteristic feathery leaves of the adult. Yarrow can also be grown from mature plant divisions (see page 5).

The beautiful white flowers grow in flat clusters on the plants, attracting butterflies and beneficial insects to your garden. Mature yarrows send out runners that will cause the plants to spread. If you don't remove the spent blooms, yarrow will also reseed itself.

Harvesting and Storage of Yarrow

Early in the season, when yarrow is in full bloom, cut the stems halfway down (above the leaf joint). Dry the leaves and flowers on the stems, then strip them off, discarding the stems. Store the dried leaves and flowers in a glass container away from heat and light. Later in the season, during the last blossoms, cut the stems all the way down to the ground.

Suppliers of Herb Seeds

Allen, Sterling & Lothrop
207-781-4142
www.allensterlinglothrop.com

Johnny's Selected Seeds
877-564-6997
www.johnnyseeds.com

Fedco Seeds
207-426-9900
www.fedcoseeds.com

Nichols Garden Nursery
800-422-3985
www.nicholsgardennursery.com

Harris Seeds
800-544-7938
www.harrisseeds.com

W. Atlee Burpee & Co.
800-888-1447
www.burpee.com

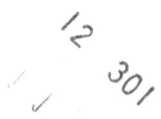